Dukan Diet

Simple And Delicious Recipes For The Dukan Diet's
Consolidation And Stabilization Phases

*(Seven-day Menu For The Second Phase Of The Dukan
Diet)*

Dwight Lamarche

TABLE OF CONTENT

Chapter 1: What Is The Dukan Diet?............................ 1

Chapter 2: The Initial Two Procedures........................ 8

Chapter 3: Breakfast Dukan Diet Recipes That Are Quick And Simple..16

Chapter 4: The Guidelines For The First Two Segments. 36

Chapter 5: The Four Segments Comprising The Dukan Diet 39

Turkey Stew 50

Chapter 6: Benefits Of The Dukan Diet 52

Chapter 7: The Dukan Diet: Getting Started 54

Chapter 8: Dukan & Other Diets 63

Chapter 9: Is It Supported By Evidence?..................73

Chapter 10: Imperceptible Fall 79

Cinnamon Spiced Latte..112

Peruvian Green Sauce 113

An Overview Of The Anti-Inflammatory Diet........116

Cherry Quinoa Cereal 118

Chocolate-Flavored Ice Cream..................................120

Grilled Spicy Shrimp 122

Mini Burgers 124

Salmon Burger..129

Simple Soufflé For Lunch...131

Yogurt-Based Dipping Sauce...133

Chapter 1: What Is The Dukan Diet?

Pierre Dukan, a French nutritionist and dietitian, developed the Dukan diet, a protein-based eating regimen. It is intended primarily as a rapid weight loss program that does not involve calorie counting or sensations of hunger. However, you are limited to 2 00 dietary options, of which 68 are animal-based and 6 2 are plant-based. This means that you can consume as much as you want as long as you stick to the list of 2 00 permitted foods.

The Guarantee

If you adhere to the rules of the Dukan diet, you could lose up to 2 0 pounds in the first week and 2 to 8 pounds per week until you reach your weight loss target, all without starving yourself. If you continue to adhere to the diet rules through the final phase, you will never regain the weight you've lost.

The Doctrine

The primary focus of the Dukan diet is protein, which contains fewer calories (8 calories per gram) than foods abundant in carbohydrates or fat. Additionally, protein has a "satiating" effect, causing dieters to consume significantly less. And because the diet restricts carbohydrate consumption (the body's preferred source of energy), your body is compelled to burn fat stores as an alternative fuel, resulting in accelerated weight loss.

Dukan vs. Atkins

According to its advocates, the Dukan diet is comparable to the Atkins diet in a number of respects. Both diets emphasize minimal carb consumption in order to induce ketosis, a metabolic state in which the body is prompted to burn fat as fuel rather than sugar. However, these two diets have significant differences:

• Fat Content - The Dukan diet includes low-fat protein sources, whereas the Atkins diet has no restrictions on saturated fats (meat lipids included) and dairy. Dr. Dukan asserts that a diet low in fat is healthier for heart health.

• Natural Foods – The Dukan diet rigorously enforces the rule of adhering to the list of 2 00 permitted foods, all of which are 2 00 percent natural. The Atkins diet, on the other hand, permits the consumption of packaged foods, bars, and smoothies.

• Calorie monitoring – as stated previously, the Dukan diet does not require calorie monitoring. During any of its four phases, there is no need to track other nutritional values. However, the Atkins diet restricts caloric consumption throughout the duration of the diet. This means that you will have to count calories from the start of the diet and throughout its duration.

• Food Options – The Atkins diet restricts vegetable consumption because devotees tend to exceed their daily carbohydrate limit, whereas the Dukan diet permits the consumption of vegetables as long as they are on the list of permitted foods.

• An Interactive, Personalized Diet Plan – The Dukan diet provides a personalized diet plan and includes online coaching support that monitors the dieter's daily progress. The Atkins regimen has no equivalent plan.

This section is not meant to be critical of the Atkins regimen. Its sole purpose is to outline the main distinctions between the two well-known diet plans as a guide for dieters.

Your Real Mass

Before beginning the Dukan diet, it is essential to determine your actual weight. Your actual weight may not be the same as your ideal or intended weight. Rather, it is the weight you can attain without sacrificing your health or struggling. Additionally, it is the weight that you can maintain without difficulty, deprivation, or a restricted diet.

On the official website of the Dukan Diet, you can calculate your actual body weight. You will be required to input specific information into their online calculator upon arrival. It will then construct a customized diet plan for you and determine your actual weight loss objective. The required details include the following:

• age • gender • average weight • desired weight • lowest weight you've ever attained • highest weight you've ever attained • heredity (genetic trends regarding weight gain) • number of pregnancies (if applicable) • bone structure

The website will send you a graph and data based on your measurements indicating which phase of the Dukan diet you should be on and for how long.

Chapter 2: The Initial Two Procedures

In a maximum of seven days, the attack procedure causes the weight-watcher to lose two to three kilograms of weight. During this phase, the weight-watcher's metabolism is prepared for the initial phase of the diet. The dieter is permitted to consume protein from 80 different food categories.

Depending on the patient's level of obesity, the schedule would vary. It can be manually adjusted or measured throughout the diet's duration. Simply put, the duration of the assault program can be adjusted accordingly.

The primary objective of the assault is to introduce a nutritious diet. The patient will consume only enough food to satisfy appetite. The greatest amount of weight is lost during this process. The body will gradually adapt to the steady rate of weight loss.

The initial days of this phase are the process's most crucial. The dieter must make concessions to his previous eating patterns in order to adopt the new routine of following the process. Among the few disadvantages of this regimen, the initial fatigue is notable. However, the condition improves within three days. The patients' fluctuating energy levels prevent them from engaging in vigorous exercise. This program necessitates three whole meals per day, which is another reason for less exercise. It makes the patient feel satisfied, which is crucial for discouraging patients from eating anything other than protein.

In addition to 2 2 2 tablespoons of oat bran per day, the following foods are recommended for the assault phase:

2 . Trimmed beef, rabbit, or veal, excluding the ribcage

Turkey and chicken without skin, as well as the wing tips

6 . lean ham, thinly sliced

8 . Liver

10 . Fresh seafood

Crabs, prawns, and other forms of crustaceans and shellfish

7. Two fresh eggs per day, preferably without the yolk

2% or less reduced-fat dairy products

Non-fructose sweeteners, spices, mustard, vinegar, herbs, onion as a spice, garlic, lemon juice only as a condiment and not as a juice drink, sugar-free ketchup and sugar-free chewing tobacco.

Occasionally, some adverse effects of the assault process do manifest.

Constipation is one of them because protein-rich diets lack fiber. The Dukan Diet requires the consumption of oat flour for this reason. However, sufficient water and wheat bran meal can rectify the issue.

Protein-rich diets can lead to respiratory difficulties, which can be remedied with water. Additionally, sugar-free chewing gels can be useful.

Protein-rich foods can induce dehydration because they stimulate kidney function. To combat this issue, the daily water intake should be increased to 2 .10 liters.

As oat bran is a required dietary component, it is recommended to consume it in the form of porridge, a yogurt counterpart, or as a component of pastries or breads.

During the assault process, both the physical and nutritional aspects must be maintained. Exercise ought to be minimal. Twenty minutes of walking is adequate.

It is observed that no improvement is discernible after approximately five days. At this stage in the process, the dieter must transition to the subsequent phase, known as the cruise phase. It is advised that the attack procedure not be prolonged.

Simple online research can help you discover additional meals to complement the recommended Dukan Diet foods.

Cruise Period

After the effective completion of the attack phase, the cruise phase would begin. At this point, approximately two pounds or one kilogram should be lost per week. The dieter would partition each meal set into two five-day portions: (i) pure protein, and (ii) a mixture of protein and vegetables. It is a challenging dietary regimen, so the dieter must be motivated. Alternating between the cuisines on a daily basis is an alternative option. This time, a similar result is obtained, although it is believed that the previous lengthy procedure had advantages. During the five-day course of the regimen, for instance, the process of skin tightening is permitted.

The elderly will observe two distinct diets: (i) a two-day protein diet and (ii) a five-day protein diet with vegetables. However, this process is slower than the previous two.

Here is a list of vegetables that should be consumed during the second phase of the aforementioned three regimens.

2 . Aubergine

2. Asparagus

6 . Artichoke 8 . Broccoli 10 . Cauliflower
6. Brussels

7. Sprouts

8. Chicory 9. Courgette 2 0. Celery 2 2 .
Leeks 2 2. Cucumber

2 6 . French beans 2 8 . Onions 2 10 .
Mushrooms 2 6. Peppers 2 7. Squash 2 8.
Salad greens 2 9. Spinach 20. Radish 22 .
Soybeans

22. Radish 26 . Tomato 28 . Sorrel 210 .
Swede 26. Swiss chard

These vegetables have substitutes if they
are unavailable. Carrots and beetroots
can be consumed in tiny amounts
alongside the aforementioned
vegetables.

At this point in the diet, the dieter may consume two tablespoons of oat bran per day.

At this point, a 6 0-minute walk is ample for physical activity.

At the conclusion of the cruise phase, the dieter should have reached his target weight. The 2 10 th day of the Dukan Diet program will have passed at this point. The anticipated weight loss during this segment of the program is 2 6 pounds or 7 kilograms, or roughly 10 kilograms during the attack phase and 2 kilograms during the cruise phase.

Chapter 3: Breakfast Dukan Diet Recipes That Are Quick And Simple

Warm the fresh egg and bacon sandwich and savor!

Smoked Salmon Omelette Baked Dukan-Style

At any phase of the Dukan diet, nothing is superior to omelletes. The technique of baking this dish in a silicone bakeware in the oven, as opposed to preparing it in a saucepan, eliminates the need for oil in this protein-packed lunch recipe. This recipe yields two portions.

Ingredients:

2 tablespoon of fresh chopped scallions

2 tbsp preserved dill

2 tablespoon of nonfat natural yogurt

2 00 grams cured salmon

6 portions fresh eggs

black pepper that has been freshly powdered

Procedure:

First, the oven must be preheated to 2 80 degrees Celsius.

Two-thirds of the fish should be coarsely chopped and added to the fresh egg mixture. The remaining salmon will be sliced into thin strips for garnishing the completed omelette.

The fresh eggs are beaten in a basin. Add the yogurt and dill.

Place the sliced fish inside. Completely combine and season with pepper.

Pour the fresh egg mixture into a silicone or metal loaf pan. This will ensure that no additional lard is required and prevent the cooked omelette from sticking to the mold.

Place the salmon segments and chives on top of the baked omellette.

Place the mold in the center rack of the oven and bake for 6 0 minutes.

This dish can be consumed during the Attack Phase or during PP days on its own. During the Cruise Phase, especially during the P+V days, you may appreciate this recipe with a salad of mixed greens and tomatoes.

2 .2 What is dukan Diet?

The Dukan diet is a daily dietary plan consisting of four small, protein-rich meals per day.The Dukan Diet is a redeveloped variant of the old Protein sparing modified fast technique that was created many decades ago to naturally treat obesity. It is a meal plan that enables 2 00 food items per day to be consumed as meals. Dr. Pierre Dukan believed that a higher protein intake would lead to weight loss, so the starting point should be a higher protein intake with maximal carbohydrate restriction. According to Dr. Dukan, protein is a dieter's friend, while carbohydrates are his adversary.

The diet eliminated all carbohydrate consumption, which was permissible on the Atkins diet.Even vegetables with minimal carbohydrate content, such as Spanish and cabbage, are not permitted at first.Unlike the Atkins plan, this diet eliminates carbs, so fried fresh eggs and pork cuts are not permitted. In place of this, the Diet consists of lean protein-rich foods. You can consume protein-rich foods such as fish, meat, nuts, and seeds, but you cannot eat carbohydrate-rich foods such as dried fruits, cakes, and bread products. According to Dr. Dukan's hypothesis, the majority of these products are manufactured artificially and have adverse effects on human health, primarily in the form of obesity, which leads to heart and blood pressure diseases.

On the course that follows, one can expect to lose at least 6 to 10 pounds of weight within a week. The plan has the maximum number of satisfied customers and clients of any diet plan available in the United Kingdom, making it the most popular diet plan available. The Diet Plan has received the highest rating from users and is expanding into new markets.

2 .2 Why Choose a Dukan Diet

There are numerous arguments that can be made in support of the Dukan Diet.

⬜ Suppose it is 6 o'clock, which is the optimal time to wake up and go to the gym for morning exercise in order to get rid of this protruding stomach. However, what if you are unable to rouse up after having slept for 10 to 6 hours following 20 hours of continuous work and having to return to the office in two and a half hours? Therefore, exercising may not be the best option for you. Therefore, you must alter your course to eliminate this issue and surmount this heavy burden. Therefore, adopting a new diet plan may be beneficial.

☐   If you visit a market, a pharmacy, or a doctor of your choosing, they may all recommend that you use certain medications, touting their benefits and presenting them as the only solution to your problems.However, the vast majority of these pills are comprised of an unnatural combination of various constituents that are not natural at all and cause you long-term harm. The most essential aspect of the Dukan Diet is that everything is 2 00 percent natural.All that is required is a change in diet and the substitution of nutritious meals for foods that are high in carbohydrates.

If we examine our daily diet, we find that it consists primarily of carbohydrates, whether in the form of bread products or fast cuisine, for example.Now, medical science has demonstrated that there is no better choice for a person than to consume protein, as it is the substance that builds up your bones and flesh. Carbohydrates, on the other hand, are required in small amounts but have no significant positive effect on a person's physique. The Dukan Diet ensures that a person always consumes sufficient protein so that all of his requirements are met and excess fat is slowly and gradually released from the body.

Proteins are composed of amino acids that are held together by strong covalent bonds between molecules. Along with flesh, this protein builds up our bones and skeleton structure. Protein, once ingested, requires more time to break down and stays in the stomach longer than carbohydrates, thereby satisfying a person's hunger for an extended period of time. In addition, a high protein intake will reduce the production of hormones that stimulate appetite.This protein comprises the majority of the Dukan Diet Plan.

☐   Carbohydrates and fats reduce our appetite for a short period of time, and their excessive consumption can cause heart problems such as high blood pressure.

☐   There are numerous plans on the market that cause a person to restrict or diet for a specific period of time. The Dukan Diet, on the other hand, does not require you to starve; rather, it requires you to change your eating patterns in order to get rid of your troublesome belly fat.

An additional advantage of adopting the Dukan diet is the availability of online documentation and CDs on the market.

The Dukan Diet is all-natural and typically consists of products that are readily available on the market and in our residences. As a result, you do not need to consult your doctor repeatedly for complete content of food, as it is readily available in your household and guidance is available online.

2 .6 The Dukan Diet Phases

The Dukan Diet consists of four main phases that cycle the consumption of various types of protein and carbohydrates. The cycle comprises of 2 00 distinct permitted foods. This theory is supported by four fundamental pillars: assault, cruise, consolidation, and stabilization.The idea behind this is to enable fat storage to be dipped into and then assist in fat metabolism, transforming the body into a fuel-burning machine.

However, some fibrous Carbohydrates are permitted in the form of various foods such as Spanish, celery, tomatoes, and broccoli. A daily exception is made for the consumption of wheat bran. The amount of its consumption may differ depending on the stage we are in.The Dukan Diet incorporates oat bran as a primary ingredient.

The Deconstruction of Four Cycles can be described as follows:

ATTACK PHASE: The attack phase is the initial phase of this diet plan, which permits a rapid weight loss of up to 7 kilograms and forces the metabolism to operate at a very rapid rate. During this phase, the dieter can choose from 68 distinct protein products. The duration of this phase is typically 2 to 2 0 days, and the dieter must consume at least 6 containers of water per day. During this phase of the regimen, very lean protein sources such as chicken, beef, fresh eggs, and fat-free dairy products are to be consumed.This phase should not be followed for longer than 2 0 days, as excess time may result in dehydration and other complications.

CRUISE PHASE: During this phase, one may add as many non-starchy vegetables as desired and an additional half teaspoon of oat bran. This phase may last several months. This phase is designed to accelerate the person's progress toward their required or desired weight by consuming three protein-rich meals per day.One can choose from 28 permitted food items that have been designated for this portion of the plan. There is also a standard for measuring the duration of this phase, which is typically calculated as 2.2 pounds of weight loss per week. No butter or oil may be used, and the user must consume copious amounts of water daily.

CONSOLIDATION PHASE: This is the third and final phase of the cycle. Every day, you may consume one portion of fruit, three to four slices of wheat bread (whole wheat bread, if available), and a small amount of cheese. Two days per week, you may consume starch in the form of rice or any other readily available grain.It is a good phase for someone who wishes to cheat, as one can have a small amount of wine 2 -2 times per week. However, on the following day, only protein should be consumed. This phase is managed specifically to prevent future mass gain. Again, water consumption is required during this phase.

STABILIZATION PHASE: The final phase of this meal plan is the stabilization phase, which aids dieters by allowing them to consume whatever they want while requiring them to adhere to a few essentials.2 -Protein must be consumed one day per week.2-Must consume oat bran daily.6 -Never stop walking for the remainder of your existence. Dr. Dukan wanted to instill the importance of a daily walk in all individuals, so he deemed it essential to include a daily walk in the final portion of this diet plan so that people could follow this rule for the rest of their lives.

2. THE VERY BEST FOOD RECIPES

Since the Dukan diet plan consists of four distinct phases, the meals and recipes to be used in each phase are distinct from one another. Comparatively, some of them contain a substantial quantity of Protein, while others contain a comparable amount. In addition, the amount of carbohydrates, oat brans, and water consumed per day or week varies according to the cycle plan.

Within the Attack Phase of the Cycle, Dukan Diet

We are aware that the first phase of the Dukan diet, the attack phase, lasts the shortest amount of time but is the most difficult to complete.The reason for this is that one must surmount the use of the majority of carbohydrates and intake of the most protein. This naturally causes difficulty for a person who was accustomed to consuming significant quantities of carbohydrates, but is now required to consume proteins. We will provide you with some recipes for this phase, but the Dukaners are welcome to add their own preferred ingredients to make these meals more enjoyable.

☐ Ginger And Chili Roast Chicken: This recipe for ginger and chile roast chicken, which can be consumed during this phase of the diet, is the tastiest and most delicious among all others. With a 20-minute preparation time and a one-and-a-half-hour cooking time, the dish is available to delight you whenever you desire. So, you have guests coming to your residence and you want to serve them the best food? This recipe will not disappoint.

Indian Spicy Omelette:Are you from India or the subcontinent and finding it difficult to adhere to the Dukan diet because you cannot give up rich or oily foods?We have a diet designed specifically for you. This piquant omelette will satisfy your cravings for heat. On days containing protein and vegetables, it may also be served with cherry potato and salad. The omelette is very light and can be consumed with a certain quantity of cheese.

Frying Steak Pizzaiola: Do you find it difficult to eliminate carbohydrates in general? Right. We provide you with space. A recipe that satisfies both your protein and carbohydrate requirements for the day. The dish can be prepared in less than 2 0 minutes.

Spanish-Style Seafood Lunch The Spanish-style seafood lunch is prepared by combining the spiciness of red chile peppers with rounded garlic cloves. It is certainly a treat during the attack phase, satisfying your low-fat demands as well as the attack phase's basic requirements. Preparation takes 10 minutes, while cooking takes between 10 and 2 0 minutes.

Smoked salmon with cream cheese: The dairy item comes last on this list.A person following this diet must ensure that their breakfast contains adequate protein and carbohydrates.

2.2)Dukan Diet During Cruise Phase

The cruise phase is the second phase of the Dukan diet, and it is the phase that brings you directly to the weight goal you established at the outset of the program.Thus, during this phase, a person must frequently and repeatedly consume specific foods. This phase includes recipes for solo protein days, protein days with vegetables, and oat bran days.

Weight-Free Yogurt: We are aware that yogurt is intended to have a high protein content and can assist a person who wishes to increase his protein intake. Frozen yogurt is available on the market, but the fat content of the varieties sold in stores, despite claims that they contain a small quantity of fat, is still quite high for someone who has a diet plan for the coming days.Therefore, the one we are introducing to you must be prepared at home, as it is comprised of protein- and carbohydrate-rich ingredients. The only additional item required is an ice cream maker, which you must have at home or the process will take several hours. With an ice cream maker, the time required for the product is only 2 0 minutes, whereas without one, it could take up to several hours. The only ingredients are 2 tablespoon of natural yogurt (10 00 grams), 6 tablespoons of jelly, and 6 tablespoons of scalding water, unless you wish to dilute it further.

Warm tandoori chicken salad: a recipe for the Protein and vegetable day.

Tandoori chicken is a ubiquitous dish served in restaurants and hotels in the Subcontinent, but the chicken referred to here is skinless and contains very little fat (almost.002 %). This can also cause the chicken to become dry, so we add cheese on top to make it less dry and more palatable. The Recipe requires only ten minutes to prepare and two to three hours to marinate. The maximum cooking duration is thirty minutes.

Chocolate Ice Cream: We are well aware that ice cream lovers cannot even conceive of abandoning them.However, the diet plan must ensure that carbohydrates are limited and proteins are increased. Consequently, we have a delight for these ice cream fans. It requires only 2 10 minutes to prepare and 2 10 to 6 0 minutes to freeze. Three fresh eggs, a touch of vanilla or another flavor of your choosing, two tablespoons of reduced-fat cocoa, and 6 10 0 grams of fat-free frays comprise the ingredients.

Oat Bran and Galette Recipe: This recipe is designed specifically for Oat Bran days and can be used as a staple. The recipe can also be prepared in large quantities and stored in the refrigerator for later use. These are the ingredients: 6 teaspoons of oat bran, 2 fresh egg whites, and 6 tablespoons of nonfat yogurt.

Chapter 4: The Guidelines For The First Two Segments.

Following the conclusion of the assault phase, the next step is the cruise phase. The average healthy weight loss per week is approximately two pounds, or one kilogram. In this case, the dieter must alternate between two sets of dietary components on five-day intervals, namely (a) five days of pure protein intake and (b) five days during which the patient consumes a mixture of protein and vegetables. Due to the duration of each interval, the alternative scheme may be too difficult for a dieter who requires a high level of motivation to execute. Therefore, a one-day rhythm may be considered as an alternative method for alternating the two food categories. Although some theories assert that a prolonged period for each interval has some advantages, the effects are comparable. Under the five-day intervals, for instance, the epidermis is allowed for shrinkage. Consequently, flabs do not develop.

The recommended pattern for older individuals is (a) two days of pure protein and (b) five days of combined protein and vegetables. Under this procedure, fats are eliminated at a slower rate than in the two other sets of intervals described in the preceding paragraph.

All three rhythms permit the following vegetables: aubergine, asparagus, artichoke, broccoli, cauliflower, Brussel sprouts, chicory, courgette, celery, leeks, cucumber, French beans, onions, mushrooms, peppers, pumpkins, salad leaves, spinach, radish, soya beans, turnips, tomatoes, spinach, sorrel, swede, and Swiss chard. Naturally, these vegetables have localized equivalents depending on location. Also permitted, but in moderation, are carrots and beets.

Increasing quantities of oat grain continue to be incorporated. Now, the dieter can consume two tablespoons per day.

For the physical component, the patient must walk at a moderate pace for thirty minutes per day.

At the conclusion of the maintenance phase, the dieter should have reached his or her objective or desired weight. At this point, the Ducan Diet program must be fifteen days into its implementation. Under the assumptions considered here, the total weight loss should be approximately seven kilograms or sixteen pounds. Five kilograms of weight loss could have been accomplished during the attack phase, and the

remaining two kilograms could have
been lost during the cruise phase.

Chapter 5: The Four Segments Comprising The Dukan Diet

Once you decide to commence this diet,
you will experience a rapid initial weight
loss. Given these results, you will
undoubtedly feel motivated to continue
the diet. Aside from that, during the
duration of the Dukan diet, the
likelihood of experiencing frustration is
minimal. First, it is prohibited to weigh
food portions, and there is no need to
calculate caloric. Moreover, the variety
of foods permitted to be consumed is
quite extensive.

The Dukan diet is readily described as a
comprehensive and highly effective

weight loss program. Its success is assured by its rigorous structure, which promises genuine results. The Dukan Diet is structured into four phases; the first two phases are recommended for weight loss, while the latter two are intended to help you maintain and stabilize your weight.

The first phase is referred to as the attack phase, and it is during this phase that you will discover the motivation to lose weight. During this phase, you will lose weight substantially and rapidly. There are at least 72 foods on the list of permissible foods. All of them have a high natural protein content, providing you with the same health benefits as other protein-based diets without the negative side effects.

In a sense, you can view this phase as the beginning of your physical conquest. Motivated by the rapid weight loss, it will be imperative that you adhere to this regimen. Regarding the duration of the attack phase, you have entire freedom to determine the duration. In general, the duration of the assault phase is proportional to the amount of weight loss desired. The average duration of the assault phase for the majority of individuals following the Dukan diet is between two and seven days.

As you've likely deduced by now, the Dukan diet is restricted to protein consumption. Fresh egg whites are the only substance with a protein content of one hundred percent. For optimal results, the permitted foods on the diet should be as close as feasible to pure proteins. As you will see in the subsequent chapters, the variety is quite extensive and includes non-fat dairy products, poultry, seafood, certain meats, and whole fresh eggs. During the assault phase, you can anticipate losing between two and three kilograms, thereby revving up your metabolism.

During the cruise phase, you are coming close to your ideal weight. During this phase, you may alternate your consumption of natural proteins and vegetables (there are 28 recommended vegetables). Generally speaking, there are NP (natural proteins) days and PV (proteins and vegetables) days. These can be alternated in order to reach the ideal weight progressively. Even though there are many vegetables to choose from, you must avoid those with a high oil content (such as avocados) and those with a high starch content (such as potatoes).

You can compute the duration of the maintenance phase based on how much weight you still need to lose (approximate calculation: 2 kg per week). As previously stated, raw or cooked consumption of non-starchy, non-fat vegetables is permitted. The only thing to remember is that the NP days and PV days alternate. This will contribute to the elimination of that excess weight, thereby aiding in weight loss. During the cruise phase, you are permitted to consume as many vegetables as you desire (from the list of recommended vegetables). You are free to consume at any time of day and create any combination that comes to mind.

The third phase is referred to as the consolidation phase, during which the body is trained to maintain its ideal weight. The intriguing aspect of this phase is that it permits the reintroduction of high-calorie foods and special occasion meals. This phase's primary objective is to prevent you from regaining weight, which is why the natural protein day remains. Typically selected on Thursday, this day is ideal for readjusting your weight, thereby preventing a rebound.

During the consolidation phase, you are permitted to consume an unlimited amount of permitted foods, which include fruits and vegetables. In addition, you may consume one portion of lamb or pork per week. This the phase in which restrictions are relaxed and enhancements are permitted.

During the first half of the consolidation phase, you may consume one portion of fruit per day; however, certain fruits, such as cherries, figs, grapes, and avocados, are still prohibited.

In addition to the fruit allotment, you may consume whole bread (2 slices per day), hard cheese (8 0 grams), and 220 grams of starchy foods per week. The celebration supper is the icing on the cake, and one per week is permitted. This special supper may include an aperitif (wine), an appetizer, a main course, and a dessert (cheese may be substituted for the dessert). It goes without saying that each course of the celebration meal is limited to a single serving. In the second half of the consolidation phase, you are permitted two portions per week of everything listed above, with the exception of firm cheese (which remains 8 0 grams). In addition, you are permitted two festive lunches.

In conclusion, the consolidation phase will prevent future significant weight gain. The problematic foods are reintroduced progressively and in a specific order in order to reduce the risk of relapse and to ensure the maintenance of your current weight. The duration of the consolidation phase is determined by the amount of weight lost. You can roughly estimate five days for every kilogram you have lost.

Stabilization is the final and fourth phase of the Dukandiet. During this phase, you may consume whatever you wish, so long as you adhere to a set of guidelines. You must sustain the protein day once per week (natural protein Thursday), consume oat bran daily (three tablespoons is recommended), and engage in physical activity for at least thirty minutes (walking, taking the stairs, refusing the elevator). Maintaining the stabilization phase for the remainder of your life will prevent you from acquiring weight again.

Thursday NP is the most essential element of the stabilization phase to remember. If you have been observant, you have likely observed that the natural proteins day has been maintained since the attack phase. This day is crucial to the Dukan diet, in case you were pondering why. By utilizing this extremely potent weapon one day per week, you can maintain your current weight for life.

In the event that you slip up and consume unhealthy foods, the NP Thursday will enable you to get right back on track. The Dukan regimen is structured so that a positive attitude is maintained throughout. There is no reason to be concerned that this diet won't work, particularly if you adhere to all of the phases highlighted in this chapter. Remember that as long as you observe the NP day, you can consume normally on the other days of the week without fear of regaining weight.

The permitted ingredients on the Dukan diet are detailed in the following chapter. Ensure that your list of recommended foods is organized and that you begin the diet as soon as possible. There is no doubt that you will be pleased with the results and glad that you chose the Dukan diet in the first place.

Turkey Stew

Ingredients

4 tablespoons of white wine

4 shallots

4 cloves of garlic

. 2 pinch of salt and pepper

10-115   lbs of turkey breast, cut into pieces

5 lb of mushrooms, cut into pieces

5-10 large carrots, cut into pieces

5-10 tomatoes, cut into pieces

5-10 tablespoon of tomato puree diluted in ¼ cup of water.

Preparation

1. Place turkey in a casserole dish and add mushrooms, carrots and tomatoes.
2. Add tomato puree, white wine, shallots, garlic cloves, basil, salt and pepper.
3. Cover the casserole dish and leave to cook on a medium heat for 60 minutes.

Chapter 6: Benefits Of The Dukan Diet

Every day, the health risks associated with being overweight or obese increase, posing significant dangers for cardiovascular disease, high blood pressure, type 2 diabetes, stroke, and even some forms of cancer. There is also the risk of premature death to consider, as well as a general decline in quality of life, when a person carries a substantial quantity of excess weight. But even if you don't have that much weight to lose, you can still see substantial improvements in your overall health indicators, not to mention how much better you'll feel about yourself when you feel and appear healthy.

Through one or more of its numerous benefits, the Dukan Diet can help you achieve your weight loss goals rapidly and with relative ease:

The rapid weight loss you will experience during the Attack Phase will be highly motivating, and the longer-term, sustained weight loss that will bring you to your target weight during the Cruise Phase will make it simple to continue.

The strict rules effectively provide a framework within which to operate, and the limited options actually make meal planning simpler. There is no need to weigh, measure, or tally calories! You decide when you are hungry and when you are full – you will learn to listen to your body's signals. You'll be cutting out all processed, fatty, sugary, and salty foods that are low in vitamins, minerals, and nutritional value.

Chapter 7: The Dukan Diet: Getting Started

The Dukan Diet is not something that can be rushed into. You must have formulated a plan in advance. Understand that consuming only protein and a small amount of oat bran for 2-2 0 days will be stressful – this is a given. Therefore, you must be mentally prepared for this. It would be ideal to begin on a weekend, or to bookend a weekend with one or two days off from work or your normal routine. This is a significant change in your life, so you need to be able to concentrate solely on yourself.

Do not plan to begin during a stressful time in your life, such as during exam week, when you have an important interview, or when a significant anniversary is approaching, particularly if it commemorates a negative event such as a divorce or a death. Such stressful circumstances will undermine your dieting efforts even before they begin. Wait until things have settled down a bit in your life.

Utilize your time judiciously by reviewing the approved food list during the Attack Phase to determine which foods you prefer. Create purchasing lists and go to the market to stock up on enough food for at least three or four meals per day for the first few days. Remember that it consists solely of protein, oat fiber, and water. Stock up on pure herbs and seasonings that you already enjoy or are interested in trying. Herb and spice mixtures typically contain additives and sugar, which are not permitted in any phase of the Dukan Diet.

Don't forget to take it easy on yourself now that you have everything you need and are prepared to commence. If you accidentally consume something that was forbidden, it's acceptable. Just brush yourself off and return immediately to following the rules. You are a human, and all humans are flawed; this is what makes life so fascinating. If you continue to make every effort, you will triumph!

There appears to be an infinite number of regimens for those wishing to lose weight. Diets that claim to be effective at eliminating excess fat are abundant among those who seek weight loss programs.

With so many regimens available, it is difficult to determine which is the healthiest. Here are some guidelines for selecting your own diet plan.

Consult a doctor

Before beginning any weight loss program, it is essential to consult with a physician. They can evaluate your medical history to determine the most effective method for weight loss. They can also help you acquire insight into potential causes of weight gain.

Secure and efficient

It is very tempting to desire rapid weight loss, but a gradual and steady approach is typically more effective. Importantly, successful weight loss necessitates a long-term commitment, so choose a program that you can adhere to.

Consider your own requirements

Your lifestyle and preferences should play a role in your diet program. Consider the diets you've attempted in the past and determine which ones worked for you. You should also consider your finances. Some weight loss programs require the purchase of supplements or participation in fitness programs.

Weight reduction character

Plans for weight loss only work if you are committed to following them. People generally fell into one of five basic weight loss categories:

The assistance seeking

Peer motivation is necessary for those seeking aid. Their ideal plan for weight loss should include a program with a strong support network where participants can share their experiences and successes. Consider a program that offers free sample dishes and recipes if you are not very good at coming up with your own plans.

The compulsive snacker

Typically very occupied with work and family, these individuals frequently eat out of habit. Small changes, such as keeping healthy foods at home instead of the customary carbohydrate-rich snacks, can benefit snackers. The majority of serial snackers will also appreciate a time-efficient plan.

The essence of liberty

These individuals are too rebellious to adhere to a precise schedule. For these individuals, weight loss should be simple and adaptable. The free-spirited individual does not believe in restricting particular food categories. They would rather regulate their diet than eliminate an entire dietary group.

The desire for sweets

People with a sweet tooth desire cakes and cookies frequently. They will require a diet plan that meticulously plans their treats. Determine which sweet treats you cannot exist without, then plan how much and when you will consume them. Additionally, consuming sweet fruits can satisfy your sweet tooth while still providing essential nutrients.

The inattentive diner

These individuals tend to multitask and are frequently too distracted to pay attention to what they are consuming. A diner who is easily distracted must learn to plan their meals meticulously. They will also value a diet consisting of foods that can keep them satisfied for an extended period of time.

Numerous individuals believe that calorie counting is the secret to weight loss. However, what the majority of individuals do not realize is that protein plays a crucial function in weight loss. Eating protein-based foods can help you lose weight because they are generally more filling than fruits and vegetables because protein is metabolized more slowly. This is the fundamental principle behind the Dukan Diet.

When protein is the primary source of energy, all lipids and carbohydrates are eliminated, resulting in accelerated weight loss. When you restrict carbohydrates in your diet, your body is forced to use stored fat as an alternative fuel source.

This diet regimen compels the body to endure ketosis. The process by which the body utilizes its own fat reserves to produce energy is known as ketosis. Since fat stored within cells is consumed, the Dukan Diet helps to sculpt the body more quickly than exercise alone.

Chapter 8: Dukan & Other Diets

What distinguishes the Dukan Diet from other protein-heavy weight-loss diets?

The differences between the Dukan Diet and protein-based fad regimens that claim to be as effective as the Dukan Diet are listed below.

In comparison to other fad diets, the Dukan Diet is sustainable and yields enduring results. Some fad diets only help you lose weight for a brief period of time before the relapse phase, during which you regain more weight than you lost.

This particular diet plan is intended to produce accelerated weight loss during the first week, followed by gradual weight loss during the succeeding days and weeks. The Dukan Diet is the only diet that facilitates rapid weight loss in a healthful manner.

The Dukan Diet is regarded safe because it does not require dieters to starve themselves. In fact, this diet plan encourages you to eat to your heart's content, so long as you consume the recommended items.

If you adhere to the Dukan Diet's many helpful guidelines, you will achieve your desired weight loss promptly. This diet plan eliminates the need to engage in any guesswork games that could compromise your diet.

Unlike other diet plans, the Dukan Diet includes a large number of straightforward recipes. Therefore, you do not need to limit yourself to consuming the same foods repeatedly.

Although you must pay a fee for access to this diet's secrets, you only need to spend a small amount of money to obtain its benefits.

These are the reasons why the Dukan Diet is more convenient and popular than other novelty diets that are currently available.

Is This Diet Safe?

Since the Dukan Diet has been featured in the media, many individuals have questioned its safety. In addition, many individuals with a fundamental understanding of biochemistry believe that ketosis is harmful to the body.

As mentioned previously, ketosis is the process by which the body is forced to consume fat due to a deficiency of carbohydrates. Some people believe that fats stored in the body's cells are crude forms of energy that have negative adverse effects.

Although side effects such as bowel movement issues, headaches, and lack of energy may be experienced by dieters during the initial phases of a diet program, these are minimal side effects caused by an individual's diet adjustment. Moreover, ketosis is not inherently harmful because it is a coping mechanism of the body during deprivation; excessive observance of this process is what is harmful to the body.

In general, the Dukan Diet is safe for the majority of people, but those with special medical conditions should consult with their doctors before beginning this diet plan. This includes diabetics and expectant, breastfeeding, or intending to become pregnant women.

Important Measures for Weight Loss

It is vital to remember that losing weight is not about consuming less, but about eating smart! The Dukan Diet is all about consuming the appropriate foods to aid in weight loss. However, in addition to consuming the proper foods, it is also essential to observe the following guidelines when following this diet plan.

Consider The Method of Cooking. It is essential to use cooking methods that do not contribute additional calories and fats to your food when preparing meals. This implies that the Dukan Diet prohibits deep-frying. You can prepare your food in a healthy manner by baking, simmering, grilling, steaming, and roasting.

Select Lean Meats. Essential to the Dukan Diet is the consumption of lean meats; therefore, when you go grocery shopping, be sure to select fat-free, high-quality meats. On the Dukan Diet, excellent sources of protein include chicken, turkey, fish, and other forms of seafood.

Exercise Regularly. Regular exercise is essential when following the Dukan Diet. Dieters are therefore required to engage in a daily 6 10 - to 8 10 -minute exercise regimen, which may consist of brisk walking, sprinting, jumping rope, jogging, and swimming. Exercise stimulates the metabolism, which enables the body to consume calories more quickly and efficiently.

Increase Your intake of water. Due to the high protein content of this particular diet plan, dehydration is a potential side effect. This is the reason why the majority of dieters who follow this diet plan experience constipation. Every day, you must consume at least two to three liters of water to be on the secure side.

It is essential to maintain good health while following the Dukan Diet, as doing so will sustain you throughout this diet plan.

Sequences of the Dukan Diet

What differentiates the Dukan Diet from other high-protein diets is that dieters must strictly adhere to the diet's phases in order to achieve significant weight loss.

Dieters who adhere to the Dukan Diet are required to observe four phases. These are listed below:

Phase of attack Phase of cruise Phase of consolidation Phase of stabilization

Each phase is designed for a particular purpose.

The first two phases are designed to help you lose the excess weight you've been bearing, while the last two phases are intended to help you maintain your ideal weight.

Below is an in-depth explanation of what you need to know about the four phases so that you can gain a greater understanding of them.

Chapter 9: Is It Supported By Evidence?

The amount of ualtu research on the Dukan Det is limited.

One study found that Polish women who followed the Dukan Diet consumed approximately 2 ,000 calories and 2 00 grams of protein per day while losing 2 10 kilograms in 8 to 2 0 weeks.

In addition, many studies have shown that other high-protein, low-carb diets have substantial weight loss benefits.

There are multiple factors that contribute to the beneficial effects of rooster on weight.

One is the increase in calories burned during gluconeogenesis, which occurs when carbohydrates are restricted and protein intake is high.

Your body's metabolic rate increases more after eating protein than after eating carbohydrates or fat, causing you to feel replete and satisfied.

In addition, protein decreases the appetite hormone ghrelin and increases several fullness hormones, causing you to eat less.

However, the Dukan Diet differs from other high-protein diets in that it restricts both carbohydrates and fat. A high-protein, low-carbohydrate, and low-fat diet.

The rationale for fat loss on a low-carbohydrate, high-protein diet is illogical.

In one study, subjects who consumed fat along with a high-protein, low-carbohydrate meal burned an average of 69 more calories than those who did not consume fat.

The initial phases of the Dukan Diet are also low in fiber, despite the requirement that one daily serving of oat bran be consumed.

2 .10 –2 tablespoons (9–2 2 grams) of oat bran contain less than 10 grams of fiber, which is a very small amount that does not contribute to the health benefits associated with a high-fiber diet.

In addition, several healthful sources of fiber, such as avocados and nuts, are excluded from the diet because they contain too much fat.

SUMMARY˙

Although no scientific studies have been conducted on the Dukan diet, evidence suggests that it is a high-protein, low-carbohydrate approach to weight loss.

Is It Secure and Durable?

The Dukan Diet's afetu has not been studied.

However, there are numerous concerns about the effects of a high protein diet on kidney and bone health.

It was once believed that a high intake of rrotein could cause kidney injury.

However, recent research indicates that high-protein diets are safe for robust children.

That ad, reorle who are prone to developing kdneu tones could see their sondton deteriorate with a very high rroten ntake.

As long as you consume high-rotaum vegetables and fruits, your bone health will not decline on a high-protein diet.

Recent research indicates that high-protein diets have a positive impact on bone health.

Prior to beginning a high-protein diet, people with kidney disease, gout, liver disease, or other serious conditions should consult a physician.

Keep in mind that the complex rules and restrictive nature of the diet may make it difficult to follow.

Although most people will lose weight in the first two weeks, the diet is extremely restrictive on the "pure protein" day.

The diet also discourages high-fat foods that may be beneficial to your health. Animal and vegetable fats make a low-carb diet healthier, more enjoyable, and simpler to maintain over the long term.

SUMMARY

The Dukan Diet is likely secure for most individuals, but those with certain medical conditions may wish to avoid it. Restrictions on high-fat foods could be detrimental to your health.

Chapter 10: Imperceptible Fall

I had a challenging upbringing. When I was only eight months old, my mother placed me on a strict diet due to neurodermitis. While other children were enjoying ice cream, I ate curds and was grateful that I was at least permitted to consume them. You would assume that due to these restrictions I would have at least been thin, but nothing could be further from the truth. As I've stated previously and will reiterate in the future, rigorous restrictions cannot positively affect your physique. I continued to search for forbidden substances with maniacal zeal. During visits with companions, I typically ate three chocolates at once and hid the wrappers from my parents.

A revolution in my adolescent consciousness occurred when I was 2 6 years old. I fell in love with my supervisor, who was nine years older than me (I was working in advertising at the time). I believed he would notice me if I just lost weight. Therefore, I decided to seek my mother's counsel. Her response did not startle me: you must starve yourself (she lost 8 8 pounds this way when she was younger and sincerely believed that this was the only way to lose weight).

And I ceased all food consumption, with the exception of the rare compulsive eating episodes that would initiate my ordeal once more. I became exceedingly thin and even did some modeling. But the hunger strike always had to be repeated, because as soon as the deprivation ended, I dove back into food – just as I did as a child with those chocolates. My weight loss did not help me attract the attention of my supervisor. However, by that time I no longer cared.

So I continued to lose weight by alternating between starvation and "eating myself sick" I believed I could maintain my weight with these methods indefinitely. Before this, I weighed 2 2 0 pounds and stood 2 710 cm tall.

My entire existence, I used food to "chase down" my problems. I frequently began gnawing whenever I encountered a problem, not realizing that this was not the solution. I did not realize that there were other methods to deal with life's difficulties until many years later. I eventually gave up my attempts to starve myself because I was too weak to withstand these harsh methods.

When I met my future spouse at age 210 , my life became relatively tranquil. The irony is that despite the absence of anxiety and concerns, I continued to consume more food and grew even larger. Prior to the nuptials (six months after we began dating), the weight had steadily increased from 2 8 8 to 2 10 8 to nearly 2 610 pounds. When we were preparing to have a baby, I was prescribed hormone pills, and after taking them, I gained enough weight that the scale read 2 92 pounds! However, I had larger things on my mind at this point, as I was finally pregnant.

What ought to have been a period of joy was filled with suffering. During the first three months of my pregnancy, I was nearly immobile due to severe pregnancy toxemia. Then, these issues disappeared, but others emerged. My weight continued to increase consistently, and my stomach ballooned to catastrophic proportions. Despite wearing my maternity girdle constantly, I already had stretch marks by the fifth month. All of my acquaintances predicted that I would have at least triplets, and even doctors did not believe that I would only have one child. After six months, I developed severe back discomfort. I must admit that I've experienced discomfort in the abdomen since I began to gain weight. I could scarcely walk, and getting out of bed and beginning to walk every morning was an ordeal. Obviously, I was terrified to even consider physical exercises. Two weeks before my delivery, I weighed 28 7 pounds! (My abdominal circumference was greater than 2 00 cm eons ago.)

I stood on scales three days after the delivery of my daughter. I was startled to see 2 96, which is nearly the same weight as before pregnancy. After reaching 2 2 0 pounds through permanent starvation, however, even this weight was not comforting, as even this weight could not be considered sufficient.

Despite the fact that a nanny was watching my child and I returned to work almost immediately, and despite the fact that it appeared I had taken every precaution to avoid postpartum depression, it followed me relentlessly. I was unable to sit ordinarily for about a month after a difficult labor. But I attempted to walk, hired a carriage, and walked three to four hours per day. Even still, after summer, autumn arrived. I was consumed by unreasonable suffering. I was nearly always in a gloomy disposition and ate more and more each day. My spouse, a highly sensitive individual, never said to me, "Stop stuffing your face!" or "Look at yourself." Occasionally, I wish he had said it at least once or twice.

My existence became a hamster wheel of child-related housework. I was operating in full automation mode. I felt degraded. I ceased reading and losing interest in virtually everything. As the size of my clothing increased, so did the size of my plates. In addition, by March I weighed 2610 pounds and wore a size 20. How did this come about? I truly do not know!

I reached a crossroads where I had to choose between doing something or giving up permanently and forgetting that I was once on the ball. Forget about mini-skirts and snug dresses. Recognize that my constant companions will be hypertension, back pain, etc. But if I issued a challenge to myself, would it be successful? Or should I not even attempt? It felt like I was at a crossroads, and I did not feel prepared to answer this question just yet. I was overwhelmed by my thoughts and options and did not know where to begin. Suddenly, I realized I needed to take the first step to at least attempt to achieve the desired result. I wanted my daughter to be proud of her mother when she grew up. I realized all of a sudden that I desired to return to myself, to cease being a parody of the old Linda. I chose to combat despite the fact that I could barely see my opponent at the time.

Now, when my thoughts carry me back to that time, I regret not having known more about what could have helped me at the time. Consequently, I had to learn from my errors and rely solely on instinct and trial and error. Constantly, I was required to invent arguments to justify why I could not, or had no right, to give up. When there is no evidence in front of your eyes, it is difficult to believe that losing 2 6 2 pounds on your own is possible. I overcame my own skepticism.

However, you are in a superior position if you are holding this book. At least you are aware that someone, somewhere, has successfully changed her life. And you believe that you are capable of doing something similar. Now, the most important factor is to strongly believe this. As someone who has gone through the process of losing weight, I will do my best to answer any queries that you may have. And many individuals who followed me have also attained my success.

The Attack Step

The assault phase is the first phase of the Dukan diet, also known as the phase of pure proteins. This phase can result in rapid weight loss, which is one of the reasons why the Dukan diet has become so popular among celebrities, and this initial effect can serve as a powerful motivator and psychological trigger to help you remain on track for further weight loss. The attack phase of the Dukan diet can last anywhere between 2 and 2 0 days, dependent on the amount of weight you need to lose. During this phase, you are also expected to walk for 20 minutes per day.

Initial Physical Response to the Attack Phase

The first day of the assault diet will prime your body for adaptation and combat. You will have access to all of the high-protein foods on the list, including numerous popular and delectable options. However, you are not permitted to consume many of the foods that you likely consume habitually without regard to their caloric content. This phase may appear overwhelming to some, and you may initially feel restricted. The solution is to take advantage of the permitted edibles and unlimited amounts allowed.

Increase your water consumption so that you consume at least 2 .10 to 2 liters of water per day. This will help you feel full, and because you will need to urinate more frequently, you will expend more calories going to the restroom. Before beginning the assault phase, ensure that you are organized and have an ample supply of permitted foods.

When you step on the scale the morning of day 2, you should be shocked by how much weight you have lost in just one day.

The Initial Two Days of Attack Phase

If you will be in the attack phase for more than one day, which is likely given that the majority of people have more than 10 pounds to lose, then you must be aware of what to expect so that you do not become derailed and lose focus. Avoid strenuous physical activity and perform only the minimum amount of required walking as well as your customary daily exercise. You are currently attempting to acclimate, so now is not the time to go to extremes. If you want the best results attainable, 20 minutes of walking is a necessity, not a recommendation.

During the first few days of the Dukan diet, you can expect to feel a little fatigued as your body adapts to this new way of eating and works assiduously to burn and flush away fat reserves. After the second day, however, you should begin to feel more energized. During the attack phase, you may experience dry mouth or bad odor; this is not cause for concern. This is your body's response to fat loss and fat metabolism. This can reduce the severity of these disagreeable side effects.

Hunger

Following the assault phase of the Dukan diet may initially leave you feeling hungry, but this only lasts a few days and is easily remedied by consuming an abundance of the permitted foods. Hunger can be the enemy of weight loss because it indicates that your body requires fuel and causes you to consume without regard for the calories and carbohydrates you're consuming. After the third day of the assault phase, you will no longer feel hungry. This is due to the increased production of ketones, which are extremely potent appetite suppressants. After three days of eating nothing but large quantities of protein, your body has less appetite, so you eat less, and the monotony of your diet prevents you from eating calories out of boredom or excitement.

Sugar Cravings

Most of us have intense sugar cravings, typically as a result of consuming excessive quantities of sugar in the past. Similar to narcotics or alcohol, sugar can be addictive, making it difficult to resist when on a weight loss program. After three days in the attack phase, you should observe that your sugar cravings have subsided and you no longer have the same attitude toward sugary foods. Because you are no longer drawn to sweet foods and sugary indulgences as you were before beginning the Dukan diet attack phase, you will begin to make healthier food choices.

Day 8 and Beyond

After three days of the assault phase of the Dukan diet, you will begin to eat less and consume less protein. Due to the lack of fiber in your diet, constipation may become a problem by the fourth day. This problem may be exacerbated if you are not consuming enough water and other fluids at this point. You should experience less frequent bowel movements, but this is not the same as constipation. Proteins contain little fiber, and fewer gastrointestinal movements result from fewer waste products and less fiber.

If you become constipated, you can add a tablespoon of wheat bran or wheat bran flakes to your daily oat bran to increase your fiber intake without increasing your carbohydrate or calorie intake. When you begin to feel constipated, you can also consume more water because this fluid will help soften your stools, making them easier to pass. In addition to helping you flush away waste fluids, drinking more water will also increase the quantity of urine you produce. Laxatives for constipation should be avoided because they can be very aggressive and cause dependence if used for extended periods.

Never skip meals and always eat within two hours of waking up.

Skipping meals can destabilize your diet and force your body into starvation mode, where metabolic rate and fat metabolism are reduced. Skipping meals causes hunger, which can contribute to the selection of high-carbohydrate, high-calorie comfort foods. If you cannot consume breakfast immediately upon waking, drink some hot water, coffee, or tea and then wait a short while before eating. However, do not delay more than an hour. You must consume something shortly after awakening to prevent your body from entering deprivation mode and maximizing the utilization of every calorie you consume.

During the Attack Phase, Are Vitamin and Mineral Supplements Necessary?

Vitamin supplements, such as a multivitamin and mineral supplement, can be advantageous, but are not required if you will only be in the assault phase for a few days. If you have more than 10 to 2 0 pounds to lose and will be in the attack phase of the Dukan diet for an extended period of time, you may wish to take supplements to ensure that your diet does not lack essential nutrients while you are on the high protein, low carbohydrate, and low fat diet. Once you begin the cruise phase and are able to alternate days of vegetable and protein consumption with days of protein consumption only, the unlimited vegetables permitted on the list should provide all the nutrients that protein sources do not.

Water, Water, Water

Throughout all phases of the Dukan diet, but particularly during the attack phase, it is essential that you consume the recommended daily amounts of water and other fluids. If you do not consume enough fluids, you will not lose as much weight and body fat as you could that day. If you do not consume enough water, your body will be unable to flush out the byproducts of fat metabolism, which will accumulate in your system. This will impede your weight loss and may even result in a life-threatening condition known as ketoacidosis if the level of waste products in your blood causes it to become too acidic.

Results from the Attack Phase of the Dukan Diet

The assault phase of the Dukan diet can produce results comparable to those of a complete fast, but without the health risks or inconveniences associated with fasting. There are no highly processed foods on the list of approved foods, and you can consume as much as you want, so you should never feel hungry. The results you see will hinge on numerous variables. The number of pounds you need to lose, your age, and even the phase of your menstrual cycle can affect the results you achieve. Additionally, hormones influence both weight loss and water retention. Dieting frequently in the past can immunize you against weight loss, and as a result, your initial fat-burning rate may be delayed. After five days of using the assault phase, most people lose between 10 and 2 0 pounds, though others may lose more or less. Your results will hinge on your specific circumstances.

The most expedient method of travel requires a predetermined destination. The same holds true for weight loss. If you already know your target weight, reaching it will be simpler and faster. This is why the Dukan diet requires you to determine your objective first, so that the diet can be tailored to your needs. The website calculator is free to use (as long as you are willing to create an account and receive a sales pitch for nutrition coaching). If you would rather not do that and are willing to put in a little extra effort, you can also calculate your ideal weight on your own.

Optimal weight

In practical terms, "ideal" refers to the desired objective that a dieter has in mind. Everyone has unique objectives.

Kate Middleton reportedly used the Dukan Diet to lose two dress sizes prior to her 202 2 wedding to Prince William of Great Britain. Other celebrities have utilized the regimen to regain their pre-pregnancy bodies. Perhaps you want something similar because you have an upcoming public event where you want to appear your best, or because your job requires a certain level of fitness.

However, the best method to determine a target weight is to consider health. How much should you weigh based on your height and age? There is no simple response to this query.

Many specialists consider the body mass index (BMI), which compares a person's weight to their height. Others contend that the BMI underestimates body fat in overweight individuals while overestimating it in slender individuals and athletes. Do not rely on online BMI calculators or individuals who claim that your waist size should be "X" inches. Each individual has unique requirements. Ask your healthcare provider what your ideal body weight should be based on your age, gender, and physical condition.

If you have a great deal of weight to lose, you should consult a doctor about diet and exercise anyway. The Dukan diet website advises those who wish to lose more than 8 0 pounds to consult a physician. Regarding exercise, the Mayo Clinic states that brisk walking is safe for the majority of individuals, but those with heart disease, asthma or other respiratory problems, diabetes, kidney disease, or arthritis should have a thorough physical examination prior to beginning such a program.

Personalizing your diet strategy

Once you have determined your objective and obtained medical certification, you can begin planning the optimal version of the Dukan Diet for yourself. Everyone on the basic diet progresses through the four phases at their own tempo, depending on how much weight they wish to lose. Paid coaching is also available to further personalize the experience and assist with completion.

Let's put Jane Doe on a strict regimen. In six months, she will make a public appearance and must lose 10 0 pounds.

She has received a clean bill of health from the physicians. According to the website for the Dukan diet, she will spend at least seven days in the Attack phase. That's one week out of six months, and she's lost five pounds. If she continues to lose a pound every three days during the Cruise phase, it will take her 2 6 10 days, or nearly five months, to shed the remaining 8 10 pounds.

Wait! She has not yet reached the finish line.

According to Pierre Dukan, dieters are at their most vulnerable now. If Ms. Doe does not strictly adhere to the diet's Consolidation phase, she will acquire weight again. How lengthy is its duration? Five days for every pound she has lost, or 210 0 days over the course of six months. The good news is that Jane will appear magnificent at her upcoming public event. Even better news is that she will also have a month to adjust to her new diet before her event. Then, she will have a reduced likelihood of regaining that weight. The Consolidation and Stabilization phases of the Dukan diet reduce the likelihood of rebounding.

Now it is time to examine the Dukan diet in detail. This diet can be followed for free, but if you are prepared to pay, online coaching makes it even simpler. For some individuals, this form of assistance is very effective. There are two categories of coaching available. Throughout the first three phases, a monthly fee is assessed for daily interactive weight loss mentoring. It requires nightly reports from you, followed by email instructions the following morning. You also receive an online "Slimming Apartment" with tips, tools, and recipes. There are available live discussion sessions, a forum, and videos.   When   you   reach   the Stabilization phase, a distinct level of paid coaching is available to assist you in maintaining your weight loss.

The Dukan Det is a low-carbohydrate, high-protein weight loss program developed in the 2 970s by a former French physician, Dr. Pierre Dukan, to assist obese individuals in losing weight. At the time, the recommended diet for weight loss consisted primarily of low-calorie, small-portion meals, which were difficult for his patients to adhere to.

The premise of the Dukan Diet is that you do not lose weight when you are hungry. It provides food lists that are permitted during various phases of the diet, with a focus on lean protein and fat-free dairy, which promote weight loss. The Dukan Diet includes four phases: Attainment, Consolidation, Maintenance, and Stabilization. The first two phases concentrate on weight loss, while the remaining two phases emphasize maintenance.

According to proponents of the Dukan Diet, you should limit yourself to four to six rounds during the first week of the Atkins Phase and two rounds per week during the Cruising Phase. Throughout the Consolidation and Stabilization phases, you will concentrate on weight management.

What Can You Consume?

The Dukan Diet permits 68 low-fat, protein-rich foods in the first phase and 6 2 non-starchy vegetables in the second.

On the Dukan Diet, the majority of calories and nutrients come from protein, which is more filling than carbohydrates and contains fewer calories than fat.2 In addition to diet, the rlan encourages physical activity, specifically walking and utilizing the stairs rather than the elevator.

What You Should Know

The Dukan Diet does not require fasting or scheduled meal times, but it does restrict certain foods to specific days. The following are the four pillars of the Dukan Diet.

The assault rhae

The attask phase sont of consuming "rure protein"-listed foods. It targets rapid weight loss.

The theory that consuming a large amount of protein-rich foods will kick-start the metabolism. However, despite the fact that protein digestion requires a few extra calories, dietitians concur that no single food can jumpstart the metabolism. Exersise san enhance it, however.

People may lose weight during this phase because reducing carbohydrate intake depletes the body of water, which may result in significant weight loss.

The assault phase typically lasts between 2 and 10 days, but players who intend to lose more than 8 0 rounds may remain in this phase for longer than 7 days.

During the race, a person may consume any of the 68 listed animal proteins. Included are lean beef, fish, chicken, fresh eggs, turkey, cottage cheese, and fat-free dairy. Options should be low in fat and free of added sugar. A reron may consume as much food as desired, and there is no calorie counting.

The diet also mandates that they consume at least 2 .10 tbr of oat bran eash dau. The high fiber content of oat bran prevents the body from breaking down or digesting most of this carbohydrate. High fiber foods assist surrress hunger.

During the at-task phase, the regimen requires a subject to consume at least 2 .10 liters (l) of water and to exercise for 20 minutes each day.

The rough rhae

The srue rhae am to gradually reduce a person's body weight by consuming 6 2 specific vegetables. Peorle can now consume all 2 00 food items on the list, though they must alternate between consuming unadulterated rice pudding and rice pudding with vegetables.

The length of the rope depends on how much weight the rider wishes to carry. It lasts for three days per pound you wish to lose.

A person may consume an unlimited quantity of low-fat proteins and nonstarchy vegetables, such as radishes, okra, lettuce, and green beans.

In the srue phase, they must consume 2 kilograms of oat bran and exercise for 6 0–60 minutes per day.

Cinnamon Spiced Latte

1 c. skim milk

1 c. water

2 /7 tsp. cinnamon

¼ tsp. instant Coffee

Directions

In a saucepan, combine the liquid ingredients and simmer over low heat. Combine cinnamon and coffee granules in a bowl. Add dry ingredients once liquids begin to simmer. Stir carefully. Once boiling, turn off the heat. Pour into a tumbler for a warm, sugary dessert drink.

Peruvian Green Sauce

Ingredients

- Chicken Stock (enough to blend)
- Salt, Pepper, Onion Powder, Chili Powder
- Fat Free Plain Yogurt (amount varies)
- Lettuce (optional)

- 2 -10 Cloves of Garlic
- 4 Green Onions
- 1 Cup of Fat Free Sour Cream
- 1 Bunch of Cilantro

Instruction

1. Combine all ingredients, season, and pour sufficient chicken stock into a blender.
2. Taste to determine if additional seasoning is required.
3. Added yogurt to reduce the heat intensity and make the sauce creamier.
4. Refrigerate for an hour before serving with uour favored rrotein or vegetables.

An Overview Of The Anti-Inflammatory Diet

Chronic inflammation has been identified as one of the underlying causes of serious diseases, such as most malignancies and heart attack. Inflammation is a natural response of the body to an infection or injury that requires healing. However, when inflammation occurs without cause, it destroys the body and leads to illness.

Chronic inflammation is brought on by excessive exposure to pollutants, stress, genetic predisposition, inactivity, and an unhealthy diet. Since diet plays a significant role in managing this condition, it is essential to learn how to choose the correct foods to reduce the risk of disease, particularly over the long term.

The Anti-Inflammatory diet is not intended to aid in weight loss or to be followed strictly. It is more of a guide to choosing the correct foods to keep the body in optimal condition. In addition to preventing inflammation, this diet offers vitamins, fiber, minerals, and other nutrients for sustained vitality.

General Dietary Anti-Inflammatory Suggestions

Try various types of cuisine at each meal.

Include as many fresh foods as possible in each meal.

Reduce your intake of fast food and processed foods.

Consume vegetables and fruits daily.

Consume daily between 2,000 and 36,000 calories. Those who are less active will require fewer calories.

6.5100% of your daily calorie intake should come from carbohydrates, 36.00% from fat, and 20% from protein.

7. Consume more water or, if not, select beverages that contain a high proportion of water, such as fruit juices and tea.

8. Purify your potable water.

Cherry Quinoa Cereal

Ingredients:

- 1 tsp of vanilla extract
- 2 tbsp of honey
- ½ tsp of ground cinnamon
- 2 cup of water
- 1 cup of dried unsweetened cherries
- 1 cup of dry quinoa

Procedure:

1. Prepare a medium-sized saucepan and set it over medium-high heat.

2. Then, add in the water, dry quinoa, unsweetened cherries, vanilla extract, and ground cinnamon.

3. Stir the ingredients together then bring the mixture to a boil.

4. Reduce the heat then place the lid on the saucepan.

5. Let it simmer for 25 to 30 minutes or until the quinoa is tender and all the liquid has been absorbed.

6. Drizzle with honey then serve.

Chocolate-Flavored Ice Cream

INGREDIENTS

1 Tsp. Vanilla essence

4 Tsp. reduced fat cocoa powder

700 g Fat free fromage frais

6 fresh eggs, separated

Granulated sweetener to taste

INSTRUCTIONS

Add fresh egg whites to a large mixing basin and whisk until stiff peaks form. Pour in the sweetener and gently combine.

In a separate basin, whisk fresh egg yolks until thoroughly combined. Then, pour into the fresh egg white mixture while gently swirling.

Incorporate the vanilla extract, cocoa, and fromage frais into the fresh egg mixture by combining.

Slowly pour the mixture into an ice cream maker and allow it to churn until soft ice cream forms.

Remove the ice cream from the machine and enjoy. Possible to freeze up to 7 days.

fresh eggfresh eggfresh eggfresh egg

Grilled Spicy Shrimp

Ingredients

For flavor mix:

1 tsp. oregano
1 tsp. thyme
1 tsp garlic powder
½ tsp. cayenne pepper

2 tsp. newly ground dark pepper 2 tsp. paprika
1 tsp. dried stew flakes
1 tsp. onion powder

Directions

When desired, peel and devein shrimp while leaving the tails intact. Put six shrimp on each skewer. In a basin, combine ingredients for the zest blend. Brush each prawn stick with lemon juice and season both sides with the flavor blend. Cook on a barbecue, rotating every 30 minutes.

Mini Burgers

Ingredients

- 2 green chili, chopped [optional]
- Chicken breast (10 00 gm), minced
- 2 fresh egg
- 4 small garlic cloves, chopped
- Oat bran (2 tbsp)
- Cajun spice mix (2 tbsp)

Direction

1. Blend chicken breast along with the rest of the ingredients in a blender until form smooth batter.
2. Shape the mixture and form burgers by using your hands.
3. Heat the griddle pan for few minutes over high heat.
4. Arrange burgers on the pan and cook until done.
5. Serve with Greek yogurt.

Thai Chicken Burgers With Spring Onion and Chive Dip

Ingredients:

For the chicken patties:

2 small piece of peeled and chopped fresh ginger

Half a red onion, chopped or spring onions

8 tablespoons of fresh coriander

700 g of cooked or leftover chicken

2 chopped garlic clove

2 roughly chopped green chili

For the dip:

4 tablespoons of fresh chopped chives

6 chopped spring onions

A splash of lemon juice

Salt

Black pepper

500 g of zero fat Greek yoghurt

Instructions:

To make the dip, simply combine all the ingredients together in a portable blender. To season the mélange to your liking. Then, transfer it to a small container, cover it with plastic wrap, and refrigerate it until use. To make the Thai patties, simply combine all the ingredients in a food processor until they are thoroughly combined.

Use your hands to shape the mixture into six miniature cakes. Lightly oil a nonstick pan, preheat it, and sauté the chicken patties over low heat until they begin to turn golden brown. As the chicken has already been prepared, they only need a few moments on each side to combine the flavors. With the Greek yogurt dipping sauce. This recipe serves only two individuals.

Salmon Burger

- 4 tablespoons fromage frais (fat-free)
- 2 teaspoon baking powder
- 2 teaspon mustard
- A few sprigs of dill, finely chopped
- 2 slice smoked salmon
- 2 fresh egg
- 6 0 grams quark (fat-free)
- 4 tablespoons oat bran

In a small basin, combine the oat bran, fromage frais, and baking powder.

Pour the combined ingredients into a round mold and bake for 5-10 minutes in a microwave oven.

After removing the loaf from the mold, cut it horizontally.

apply mustard on one side of the sliced bread, then apply quark on the other side. Distribute the dill evenly and then arrange the cured salmon on top.

5.Top the burger with the remaining half of the bread and savor your delicious meal.

Simple Soufflé For Lunch

YoIngredients:

- Sea salt
- Black pepper
- 2 Tbsp. minced fresh parsley
- 8 large fresh eggs (whites only)
- 6 Tbsp. fat-free sour cream
- 2 Tbsp. oat bran

Method:

1. Preheat the oven to 450 °F.
2. Grease 4 little ramekins and set aside.
3. Mix the fresh egg whites with the sour cream, oat bran, and seasonings.
4. Place the mixture into the ramekins.
5. Place in the oven to bake for 60 minutes.
6. When serving, decorate with fresh parsley.

Yogurt-Based Dipping Sauce

Ingredients:

- 2 Tbsp. minced fresh parsley
- Pinch of dried cumin
- Pinch of dried thyme
- Salt
- Black pepper
- 6 Tbsp. fat-free plain Greek yogurt
- 6 Tbsp. fat-free sour cream
- 2 Tbsp. lime juice
- 2 Tbsp. lime zest

Method:

1. In a mixing bowl, combine all of the listed ingredients.
2. Refrigerate this sauce in an airtight container until ready to use.

www.ingramcontent.com/pod-product-compliance
Lightning Source LLC
Chambersburg PA
CBHW060511030426
42337CB00015B/1840